PERIMENOPAUSE DIET COOKBOOK FOR BEGINNERS

An Easy, Step-by-Step Guide to Deal with Irregular Menstrual Cycle, Hot Flashes, Rapid Weight Gain, Hormonal Changes

Sarah Jordan LD, CCN

COPYRIGHT PAGE

The information and recipes in PERIMENOPAUSE DIET COOKBOOK FOR BEGINNERS: An Easy, Step-by-Step Guide to Deal with Irregular Menstrual Cycle, Hot Flashes, Rapid Weight Gain, Hormonal Changes are not meant to replace professional medical or nutritional advice and are provided solely for educational reasons. The author and publisher disclaim all liability for any harm that may come from following the advice in this book. Before making any modifications to one's diet or beginning a program to lose weight, it is recommended that the reader seek the advice of a healthcare provider or nutritionist.

Table of Contents

Chapter 1: Perimenopause: Overview

The transition into and through perimenopause is a time of profound complexity and change for women. This time in a person's life is marked by a change in their hormone levels and the beginning of the end of their ability to have children.

Perimenopause is more than just a professional term; it's a complex interplay between a woman's body and her mind as it goes through a series of physiological and psychological changes. Imagine a symphony in which estrogen, the conductor of the reproductive orchestra, starts to change the tempo, causing a symphony of symptoms that affect both one's physical and mental health.

Perimenopause is characterized physiologically by irregular menstrual periods, a notable change from the regular predictability of younger years.

Hot flashes are like unpredictable sparks that put out the steady flame of normalcy, forcing women to deal with unexpected increases in body temperature and nocturnal sweats that can ruin an otherwise peaceful night's sleep. However, perimenopause has larger emotional repercussions than just the physical changes that occur. Mood swings are an unwanted companion that can turn a normal day into a roller coaster of emotions.

The transition through perimenopause is not a straight line; rather, it resembles a winding river.

Changes in hormone levels cause not only physical but also mental health difficulties. When estrogen levels drop, noticeable changes occur in the brain, and the once-lucid thinker may struggle with periods of forgetfulness or brain fog. It's a phase of adaptation, needing resilience and self-awareness.

To make sense of the perimenopausal experience, we need to look at it from more than just a professional perspective; we need to be sympathetic to the whole person. Successfully navigating this period requires an appreciation for the transformation, a recognition of the inherent value in the natural ups and downs of life. It's a period of self-discovery, an opportunity to reinvent one's relationship with age and women. The transition through perimenopause is more than simply a physiological process; it is also a story about the power of the human spirit to endure and even thrive in the face of tremendous change.

Why Knowledge is Power

Awareness in the context of perimenopause is crucial because it acts as a compass to help women navigate the complex journey of change that they face. With this enlightenment, individuals are more equipped to handle the twists and turns that come with this period of transformation. At its foundation, awareness breaks down the taboos around women's health issues, paving the way for more in-depth discussions about the physical and mental challenges of perimenopause.

To begin, there is no better catalyst for preventative health care than education. Women can improve their chances of receiving an early diagnosis and appropriate treatment by being familiar with the symptoms of perimenopause and discussing them openly with their healthcare providers. In addition to improving quality of life during perimenopause, this also paves the way for a healthier aging process in the years to come.

Second, education eliminates prejudice against women going through the menopause. It promotes a change in cultural narratives, making it easier for people to relate to one another and work together. As a result of the taboo being broken, women feel more comfortable reaching out for help, which strengthens bonds of friendship and solidarity during a potentially trying period.

Moreover, awareness is a vital resource for psychological health. Women benefit from having their perimenopausal mood swings and cognitive shifts put in context by learning more about this normal phase; this makes them feel more at ease and more accepting of themselves. It makes the transition into menopause much less of a mystery and less of a cause for anxiety.

Perimenopause education promotes gender parity because it draws attention to the specific health concerns that women confront and encourages action to alleviate those concerns. Through increased awareness and discussion, a more accepting and nurturing work atmosphere may be created for women going through perimenopause.

In essence, the value of consciousness in perimenopause is transformational. Understanding the biological process of femininity is important, but so is encouraging women to be comfortable in their own skin, teaching them to bounce back from adversity, and creating a society that celebrates women's strength at every stage of life.

Demystifying Perimenopause

The transition from perimenopause to menopause is complex, including a series of subtle but noticeable physiologic changes. This period covers several years and is marked by irregular menstrual cycles and hormonal variations, notably a drop in estrogen levels. As a continuous rather than discrete point, it highlights the multifaceted nature of this process of metamorphosis.

Hormonal fluctuations, with estrogen playing a leading role, are at the core of perimenopause. When estrogen synthesis decreases in the ovaries, menstrual cycle disruptions and other physiological changes ensue. Changes in estrogen and progesterone levels affect the reproductive system and other organs as well, leading to a wide range of symptoms in the years leading up to menopause.

Perimenopause often begins in the late 30s or early 40s, however this age range is not fixed in stone. However, not all women experience this chronological break at the same time.

Each woman going through perimenopause will have her own unique set of signs and symptoms, making the experience of this transition both personal and unpredictable.

A change from the normal menstrual cycles of childhood ushers in an era of unpredictability. The sudden and powerful waves of internal heat known as hot flashes are disruptive to everyday life and can even dampen the peace and quiet of sleep if they occur at night.

The emotional topography of perimenopause is likewise complex, typified by mood swings and shifts that traverse delight, frustration, and reflection. Emotional instability becomes an unexpected companion, forcing women to negotiate a variety of experiences that may be unfamiliar and unpleasant.

Perimenopause includes both psychological and physiological changes. Disruptions to a good night's sleep can have a negative effect on health in general. Skin elasticity changes, weight gain/loss, and libido swings are a few more potential outward signs.

Collectively, these symptoms produce a multifaceted experience that serves as a reminder to women that perimenopause is more than just a biological transition; it is a comprehensive metamorphosis that involves the body, the mind, and everything in between.

Hormonal Changes in Perimenopause

Hormonal changes in a woman's body are an integral part of the journey through perimenopause. Estrogen, the orchestra's chief conductor, assumes center stage at this time.

Hormonal shifts begin when the ovaries gradually lower estrogen production during perimenopause. The fluctuating nature of this reduction contributes to the wide range of perimenopausal symptoms, some of which can be rather surprising.

Progesterone, like estrogen, is a crucial hormone in a woman's reproductive system, and its levels fluctuate throughout perimenopause. The hormones estrogen and progesterone, which work together to regulate menstruation, are thrown off balance. Among the many symptoms associated with this time of change is menstrual irregularity, which might be caused by this imbalance.

These hormonal changes affect tissues and organs all across the body, not only the reproductive system.

For instance, estrogen is essential for proper cognitive function, cardiovascular health, and bone density. Women may experience shifts in various areas when their levels fluctuate, highlighting the far-reaching influence of perimenopausal hormonal dynamics. The key to successfully managing the many facets of perimenopause and maximizing well-being during this transitional time is an awareness of and ability to adapt to these changes.

Perimenopause and Reproductive Health

During perimenopause, a woman's estrogen levels, the major hormone controlling her reproductive system, fluctuate in complex ways. Shorter or longer periods and irregular ovulation might result from the ovaries gradually decreasing estrogen production, which is reflected in the menstrual cycle.

Perimenopausal symptoms including hot flashes, mood swings, and altered sleep habits can be traced back to these hormonal fluctuations. The complex interplay between estrogen's cyclical rise and fall, and the delicate symphony of physiological and psychological well-being, demands a comprehensive knowledge.

Progesterone, the reproductive melody's accompanist, also goes through considerable shifts with estrogen throughout perimenopause. Progesterone, a hormone normally connected with the second part of the menstrual cycle, is now dancing with the unpredictable hormonal changes of perimenopause.

Reproductive harmony is broken as the carefully regulated equilibrium between estrogen and progesterone is thrown off. Infertility issues might arise as a result of hormonal disruptions including missed or irregular periods or even complete anovulation.

In addition to helping you make sense of your perimenopausal symptoms, knowing how your progesterone levels vary is essential for managing any reproductive difficulties you may have.

The aggregate influence of estrogen variations and progesterone shifts during perimenopause goes beyond the immediate area of monthly abnormalities. The importance of reproductive health for women's overall health and happiness is highlighted. When fertility was previously abundant, it is now complicated by irregular ovulation and shifting menstrual cycles. The route towards conception may become more complex, urging women to negotiate these changes with awareness and, when required, seek help in managing their reproductive health throughout perimenopause.

Chapter 3: Managing Symptoms of Perimenopause

Symptom management during perimenopause calls for an all-encompassing strategy that may help women through the many difficulties they may confront. Symptom relief and general improvement are prioritized through personalized approaches because of the complexity and uniqueness of the perimenopausal experience.

To begin, honest dialogue is necessary. Insights into women's experiences can be gained by encouraging them to give voice to their physical and emotional problems. Because of this, we may treat patients' symptoms with greater care and compassion.

Management of symptoms is often aided by attending to hormonal shifts. Hormone treatment is an option for some women since it can restore a healthy ratio of estrogen to progesterone in their bodies. However, hormone treatment is pursued only after thorough assessment of the individual's health, medical history, and the unique form of symptoms.

Nutritional counsel is crucial, stressing a balanced diet rich in nutrients that support bone health, cardiovascular function, and general vigor. If you don't get enough of either calcium or vitamin D from your diet, you can benefit from taking a supplement. In addition, taking omega-3 fatty acids and drinking enough of water can help with inflammation management and reducing the severity of some symptoms.

As part of a more comprehensive strategy, engaging in regular physical activity is advocated. Exercise not only helps control weight and maintain cardiovascular health but may also ease mood swings and improve sleep quality. The key to long-term adherence is making exercise recommendations that are specific to an individual's current fitness level and personal preferences.

Emotional distress can be treated with cognitive-behavioral techniques. Women can better control mood swings and lessen stress's negative effects by practicing stress management strategies like mindfulness and relaxation exercises.

A medical professional offers constant care and monitoring. Checkups at regular intervals allow for the monitoring of symptom development, the modification of treatment plans as needed, and the identification of any new issues that may arise. When women are included in the decision-making process, they are better able to control their symptoms during the perimenopausal transition.

Perimenopause and Mental Health

The psychological effects of perimenopause are the result of a complicated interaction between a woman's changing body, her shifting emotions, and her life as a whole. Neurotransmitter activity is affected by hormonal variations, notably the fall in estrogen, which can lead to mood swings, impatience, and a heightened susceptibility to stress. These changes in hormone levels may have an effect on serotonin, which might have consequences for mood control.

Psychosocial variables also have a role in perimenopausal women's emotional well-being. Knowing that your reproductive identity is shifting as you age might make you feel sad, confused, or reflective. Mental health might be further impacted by the emergence of body image problems. To successfully navigate these complex feelings, one must take into account not only the physiological but also the psychological aspects of perimenopause.

Alterations in cognition, such as "brain fog" or memory lapses, can have an effect on one's mental health as well. These shifts are usually rather small and reversible, yet they can nonetheless lead to unpleasant emotions like irritation or worry. The psychological burden can be lessened if women are educated about the normality of these cognitive changes and given tools for controlling them.

It's important to keep in mind that not every woman goes through the same exact thing throughout perimenopause. While some women may experience a surge of joy and independence, others may struggle with darker feelings. Creating a friendly atmosphere that embraces the range of experiences is crucial.

From a mental health viewpoint, treatments may include counseling or therapy to give a space for women to explore and process their feelings. Whether it's dealing with stress or adapting to a shift in how you see yourself, cognitive-behavioral tactics might be useful. Friends, family, and community groups may all be great sources of emotional reinforcement.

Overall, a holistic approach to perimenopausal mental health include learning about the interplay between biological and psychological aspects, offering support and education, and developing individualized plans of care.

A more pleasant and resilient experience throughout this pivotal life stage may be achieved by empowering women with information and promoting a caring and inclusive discussion surrounding mental health.

Perimenopause and Emotional Well-being

During perimenopause, a woman's emotional health can take on a variety of forms, depending on her unique circumstances. Hormonal swings throughout this time period are a known contributor to erratic emotional states.

Some women may experience this as increased irritability, mood swings, or sensitivity to stress. It's crucial to remember that experiencing perimenopause and its effects on one's mental health is a uniquely personal journey, with a wide range of possible outcomes.

The psychological effects of aging and the shifting sense of reproductive identity are important factors in emotional health. Introspection, reflection, and, in rare situations, feelings of loss or doubt might be prompted by the realization that one's reproductive years are coming to an end. A sympathetic and supportive approach that recognizes the variety of women's experiences is necessary for navigating these emotional complexities.

Perimenopausal women may experience a decrease in emotional well-being if they are preoccupied with their bodies. Women may find it difficult to accept their changing bodies when they experience weight gain or loss and a loss of skin suppleness. Building emotional strength requires promoting a constructive and accepting outlook on these physical transitions.

Despite the difficulties, perimenopause may be a time of increased freedom and confidence for many women. The change might prompt introspection, personal development, and the acceptance of previously unknown facets of one's identity. Emotional well-being may be enhanced by developing resilience and coping mechanisms, such as mindfulness and stress management.

The importance of social support to one's mental health cannot be overstated. Sharing with loved ones or those in similar situations might help you feel less alone, acquire perspective, and gain perspective on your situation. It's also important to be completely honest with your healthcare professionals about your emotional problems so that you can work together to find the best course of treatment, whether that's dietary changes or psychotherapy.

Recognizing the range of emotions experienced during perimenopause, helping people develop a healthy self-perception, bolstering their resiliency, and opening lines of communication are all important ways to promote emotional health. Women might feel more confident and flexible as they traverse this transitional period if they take a comprehensive approach to their emotional well-being.

Navigating Relationships During Perimenopause

Communication, empathy, and mutual support are essential tools for navigating relationships during perimenopause. The hormonal and emotional shifts that come with this era can have far-reaching consequences for a person's close personal and family ties.

Honest and open dialogue is essential. It's important for women going through perimenopause to be able to open up to their loved ones about how they're really feeling, what symptoms they're having, and what they need. Also, it's important for loved ones to listen carefully and empathize, so that problems may be expressed freely.

To arm oneself with knowledge is to arm oneself with strength. It's important for women and their partners to gain a shared understanding of the perimenopausal transition. Information sharing may clear up confusion, calm fears, and forge a unified front against the obstacles of this time of change.

Mood and emotional swings are normal throughout the transition to menopause. Spouses and relatives should respond to these shifts with understanding and tolerance. Supportive environments may be created when people are aware that these emotional fluctuations are usually only transient and related to hormone changes.

During perimenopause, it is usual for women to experience shifts in libido and sexual desire. Having frank discussions about these shifts is essential. To stay emotionally connected and meet each other's needs, couples may need to try something new.

Family and friends may be helpful by taking an active role in adopting healthier habits that contribute to improved health. Taking part in physical activities as a family, changing to a better diet, and making your house a more pleasant place to be are all good examples of this.

Seeking the help of a couples therapist or counselor is highly recommended if navigating relationship dynamics becomes difficult. With professional help, couples can feel safe voicing their problems and working together to find answers.

For women with children, addressing the changes occurring during perimenopause to family members helps develop understanding and patience. When loved ones are included in transition planning, everyone works together to foster a positive atmosphere.

Couples and families may manage the challenges of perimenopause by encouraging open dialogue, empathy, and flexibility. Understanding that this is not an isolated ordeal can help build bonds and make for a smoother ride as you navigate this time of change.

Chapter 4: Impact of Perimenopause on Fertility

There is a complicated interplay between biological changes and possibly emotional factors between a woman's fertile and perimenopausal years.

Fertility decreases gradually in premenopausal women. Less eggs are produced by the ovaries, and those that are produced may be of inferior quality. Because of menstrual cycle changes and ovulation swings, this might make it difficult to conceive. Women in this stage of life who are trying to conceive should be aware of these shifts and seek advice from healthcare practitioners or fertility experts if they run into any challenges.

For practical family planning purposes, knowledge of the correlation between perimenopause and decreased fertility is crucial. The time it takes a woman to conceive may lengthen, and she may be more likely to miscarry, if she tries to get pregnant.

This is why it's so important for couples to talk openly about their reproductive wishes. Family planning, fertility preservation, and the use of assisted reproductive technologies are all areas in which it may be beneficial to seek expert guidance.

Emotionally, handling reproductive issues during perimenopause can be tough. The desire for children may endure, and coming to grips with the shifting landscape of reproductive possibilities can provoke complicated emotions. If you need a safe space to talk about your thoughts and consider your alternatives, reaching out to healthcare providers, counselors, or support groups can be a great resource.

Fertility decreases significantly during perimenopause, although it does not stop altogether until menopause is achieved. When a woman has not had a menstrual cycle for 12 months, the diagnosis is menopause. Up until then, conception is still possible, but at a lower probability.

A woman's reproductive path includes both fertility and perimenopause. Individuals and couples experiencing fertility issues during this transitional period would benefit greatly from more self-awareness, more candid communication, and access to expert support. Perimenopausal women's biological and emotional fertility needs need to be met for optimal health and decision-making.

Fertility Challenges Associated with Perimenopause

When a woman reaches the perimenopausal stage, she faces fertility issues as a result of the confluence of biological changes and emotional concerns that influence family planning. Predicting ovulation can be difficult for couples trying to conceive when one partner experiences the irregular menstrual periods typical of perimenopause. As women age, their egg quality and quantity decrease, making pregnancy more challenging and increasing the chance of chromosomal abnormalities and subsequent loss.

Due to hormonal changes, ovulatory failure is widespread during perimenopause, further complicating attempts to conceive. As a result of age-related decline in ovarian reserve, fewer eggs are viable, making pregnancy more difficult.

Individuals and couples who wish to start a family may experience significant emotional strain while confronting fertility issues during perimenopause. This understanding may cause a range of feelings, including sadness, anger, and loss.

Putting one's mental health first is essential, and reaching out for help from healthcare providers, counselors, or support groups can make it easier to deal with difficult feelings. It usually takes a holistic strategy to solve reproductive problems.

Options, such as assisted reproductive technologies (ART) and fertility preservation techniques, can be better understood after consulting with a reproductive endocrinologist or fertility expert. Adoption and surrogacy are two alternate routes to parenting that couples may consider.

It's important to remember that perimenopausal women often have difficulties with reproduction. A more educated and empowered journey through this difficult and emotionally charged time of life is facilitated by open communication with healthcare experts, emotional support, and considering various family-building alternatives.

Family Planning Discussions Pertaining to Perimenopause

It is important for women and men going through perimenopause to talk about family planning. Partners lay the groundwork by freely discussing their thoughts, hopes, and fears in relation to starting a family. This includes talking about having more kids, when those kids could come along, and how perimenopausal changes might play a role in those choices.

It's crucial to have a firm grasp of the physiologic shifts that occur during perimenopause. Informed decision-making is fostered when both spouses are aware of potential emotional consequences, difficulties with conception, and menstrual cycle irregularities.

In order to cooperatively form objectives during perimenopause, conversations on family planning should entail shared decision-making that takes into account individual views, wishes, and concerns.

It's critical to investigate a range of reproductive choices. Natural conception, ART, adoption, and surrogacy are all options for couples. Couples may make decisions that are in line with their beliefs and circumstances if they have a thorough understanding of the options accessible to them and their consequences.

Discussions on family planning should take emotional factors into account. It's important to recognize the loss or sadness that comes with reaching the end of your reproductive years. When dealing with the emotional components of these discussions, seeking support from healthcare experts or counselors might be helpful.

Couples may better negotiate the complexity of perimenopause and make decisions that match with their vision for the future if they approach family planning talks with openness, understanding, and a desire to explore possibilities.

Career and Professional Challenges Associated with Perimenopause

Navigating career and professional challenges during perimenopause can be a complex journey, as women contend with physical and emotional changes while managing the demands of the workplace. Communication and self-care become pivotal strategies for coping with these challenges.

One significant professional challenge is managing symptoms such as hot flashes, mood swings, and fatigue while at work. Open communication with supervisors and colleagues can create a supportive environment. Sharing one's experience with trusted coworkers may lead to increased understanding and accommodations, such as flexible work hours or adjustments to the office environment.

Another challenge is the potential impact of cognitive changes, often referred to as "brain fog," on job performance. Strategies for coping with these changes include prioritizing tasks, breaking them into smaller, manageable steps, and utilizing tools like calendars or reminders. Communicating with supervisors about potential adjustments to workload or responsibilities may also be beneficial.

Emotional well-being is integral to professional success. Coping with stress, anxiety, or mood swings may involve adopting self-care practices both at work and in personal life. Incorporating mindfulness techniques, taking short breaks, or finding a supportive network within the workplace can contribute to emotional resilience.

Striking a balance between career aspirations and personal well-being is essential during perimenopause. This may involve reassessing priorities, setting realistic goals, and recognizing the value of self-care. Seeking mentorship or guidance from others who have navigated similar challenges in their careers can provide valuable insights.

Additionally, workplaces that prioritize employee well-being and offer supportive policies can significantly contribute to coping with professional challenges during perimenopause. Flexible work arrangements, employee assistance programs, and awareness campaigns can foster a culture of understanding and support.

Ultimately, the key to coping with career challenges during perimenopause lies in a proactive and communicative approach. By openly addressing symptoms, seeking necessary accommodations, and prioritizing self-care, women can continue to thrive in their professional lives while navigating the transformative journey of perimenopause.

Preventive Health Measures for Perimenopause

During perimenopause, it is especially important to take care of your bones since falling estrogen levels are linked to decreased bone density and an increased risk of osteoporosis. Weight-bearing workouts, such as walking or strength training, and a balanced diet high in calcium and vitamin D are crucial for bone health.

Bone density tests should be performed often, especially for individuals at higher risk, because the data gleaned from them can be used to intervene and prevent issues before they become severe. Taking these preventative measures is crucial for maintaining bone health and avoiding osteoporosis's side effects.

Because hormonal changes during perimenopause can affect lipid profiles, increasing the risk of cardiovascular disease, cardiovascular health becomes increasingly important at this time. Adopting a heart-healthy diet, engaging in regular exercise, and managing stress are all essential components of cardiovascular health.

Preventive care measures such as checking blood pressure, cholesterol, and weight are crucial. Women should also talk to their doctors about the possible connection between hormone medicines and cardiovascular risks, so that they may make the best option for their heart health.

Awareness of cancer risks, especially breast and cervical malignancies, rises during perimenopause.

Routine screenings, such as mammograms and Pap smears, are an important part of preventative healthcare. For an accurate risk assessment, knowledge of one's own and one's family cancer history is essential.

The chance of developing cancer can be lowered by adopting a healthy lifestyle, which includes eating well, being physically active, and not smoking. To ensure that women are able to make their health a priority through the use of screenings and prevention strategies, interactions with healthcare professionals should go beyond breast and cervical cancer detection.

Chapter 5: Nutrition and Perimenopause Diet

Particularly during the transitional perimenopause period, one's food and nutrition play crucial roles in supporting general health. Dietary decisions can have a major influence on symptom management and long-term health as the body responds to hormonal changes and altering metabolic demands.

During perimenopause, you need more than ever to eat a healthy, nutrient-dense diet. The need of calcium and vitamin D for bone health increases at this time, since issues like osteoporosis may become more widespread. Dairy products, green leafy vegetables, and fortified meals can all help with this.

Fatty fish like salmon and flaxseeds are good sources of omega-3 fatty acids, which may help with inflammation management and cardiovascular health as you go through your menstrual cycle.

In order to control one's weight and keep one's energy levels up, one must eat a diet that includes a healthy amount of carbs, proteins, and fats. A nutritious and balanced diet includes whole grains, lean meats, and healthy fats from foods like avocados and almonds.

The importance of staying hydrated in the management of symptoms like hot flashes and in maintaining general health is often underestimated. Getting enough water might ease some of the discomforts of perimenopause by helping the body continue functioning normally.

Because they can worsen symptoms like irritability and insomnia as well as affect general health, processed foods, caffeine, and alcohol should be used with caution.

Different people have different nutritional needs, so it's best to go to a doctor or a qualified dietitian to get advice that's specific to you. Women going through perimenopause can improve their health and well-being by placing a premium on nutrition and making educated dietary decisions.

Foods to Eat on the Perimenopause Diet

Dietary priorities during perimenopause should be on nutrient-rich foods that help maintain general health and meet the unique nutritional demands of this time. The following are examples of important food groups to include in a diet during perimenopause:

Calcium-Rich Foods

- Dairy products (yogurt, milk, cheese)

- Leafy green vegetables (kale, broccoli, collard greens)

- Fortified plant-based milk (almond, soy, or rice milk)

- Tofu and fortified tofu products

Vitamin D Sources

- Fatty fish (salmon, mackerel, tuna)

- Egg yolks

- Fortified foods (certain dairy and plant-based milk, orange juice, cereals)

Iron-Rich Foods

- Lean meats (chicken, turkey, fish)

- Legumes (beans, lentils, chickpeas)

- Dark leafy greens (spinach, kale)

- Iron-fortified cereals and grains

Omega-3 Fatty Acids

- Fatty fish (salmon, trout, sardines)

- Chia seeds and flaxseeds

- Walnuts

- Algal oil (plant-based source of omega-3s)

Whole Grains

- Quinoa

- Brown rice

- Oats

- Whole wheat products (bread, pasta)

Protein Sources

- Lean meats (chicken, turkey)

- Fish and seafood

- Plant-based protein (tofu, tempeh, legumes, and beans)

Fruits and Vegetables

- A variety of colorful fruits and vegetables provide essential vitamins, minerals, and antioxidants.

Fiber-Rich Foods

- Whole grains

- Legumes and beans

- Fruits and vegetables

- Nuts and seeds

Healthy Fats

- Avocado

- Olive oil

- Nuts and seeds

It is important to eat a wide variety of foods, not only those listed above. In order to construct a tailored perimenopause diet plan that satisfies nutritional demands and addresses specific problems, it is important to pay attention to portion sizes, remain hydrated, and consider talking with a healthcare expert or a registered dietitian.

Foods to Stay Away From or Limit on the Perimenopause Diet

While there's no one-size-fits-all approach to dietary advice during perimenopause, some women may find it advantageous to limit or avoid particular foods to manage symptoms and improve general health. Here are a few things to think about:

Caffeine

While moderate caffeine intake is generally considered safe, some women may find that reducing caffeine helps alleviate symptoms like insomnia, anxiety, or hot flashes. Caffeine is found in coffee, tea, chocolate, and some sodas.

Alcohol

Excessive alcohol consumption can interfere with sleep patterns, contribute to weight gain, and exacerbate mood swings. Moderation is key, and some women may choose to limit or avoid alcohol during perimenopause.

Sugary Foods

Processed sugars can contribute to weight gain and exacerbate mood swings. Limiting the intake of sugary foods and beverages can help manage energy levels and support overall health.

Highly Processed Foods

Highly processed foods, often high in unhealthy fats, sugars, and additives, can contribute to inflammation and may negatively impact overall well-being. Opt for whole, minimally processed foods whenever possible.

Salty Foods

Excess salt can contribute to bloating and may impact blood pressure. Processed and packaged foods often contain high levels of sodium, so it's advisable to limit the intake of these items.

Spicy Foods

For some women, spicy foods can trigger or worsen hot flashes. Pay attention to individual tolerance levels and adjust the intake of spicy foods accordingly.

Fried and Fatty Foods

High-fat and fried foods may contribute to weight gain and negatively impact heart health. Choosing healthier cooking methods, such as baking, grilling, or steaming, can be beneficial.

Dairy (for Some)

Some women may experience an increase in lactose intolerance or sensitivity to dairy during perimenopause. If dairy is causing digestive issues or discomfort, alternatives like lactose-free products or fortified plant-based options can be considered.

Excessive Red Meat

While lean meats are a good source of iron and protein, excessive consumption of red meat may be associated with health issues. Consider incorporating plant-based protein sources and lean meats in moderation.

It's worth noting that people have different reactions to different meals. The best way to figure out which foods cause an adverse reaction in you is to keep a food diary and pay attention to how various meals affect your symptoms. To make sure nutritional needs are satisfied and dietary adjustments are in line with individual health objectives, it is best to speak with a healthcare practitioner or a qualified dietitian before making any major alterations to one's diet.

Chapter 6: 100+ HEALTHY PERIMENOPAUSE DIET RECIPES YOU SHOULD TRY

PERIMENOPAUSE DIET BREAKFAST RECIPES

Chia Seed Pudding with Berries:

Ingredients

2 tbsp chia seeds

1 cup almond milk

1/2 tsp vanilla extract

1/2 cup mixed berries (blueberries, strawberries, raspberries)

Preparation

Mix chia seeds, almond milk, and vanilla extract in a bowl.

Refrigerate overnight.

Top with mixed berries before serving.

Nutritional Information (per serving)

Calories: 200

Protein: 5g

Fiber: 10g

Avocado and Smoked Salmon Toast:

Ingredients

1 slice whole-grain bread

1/2 avocado, mashed

2 oz smoked salmon

1 tsp lemon juice

Preparation

Toast the bread slice.

Spread mashed avocado on the toast.

Top with smoked salmon and drizzle with lemon juice.

Nutritional Information (per serving)

Calories: 300

Protein: 15g

Healthy Fats: 18g

Greek Yogurt Parfait:

Ingredients

1 cup Greek yogurt

1/4 cup granola

1/2 cup mixed berries

1 tbsp honey

Preparation

Layer Greek yogurt, granola, and berries in a glass.

Drizzle with honey before serving.

Nutritional Information (per serving)

Calories: 250

Protein: 20g

Fiber: 5g

Spinach and Feta Omelette:

Ingredients

2 eggs

1 cup fresh spinach, chopped

2 tbsp feta cheese, crumbled

Salt and pepper to taste

Preparation

Beat eggs and season with salt and pepper.

Cook spinach in a pan until wilted, then add eggs.

Sprinkle feta on top and fold the omelette.

Nutritional Information (per serving)

Calories: 220

Protein: 18g

Calcium: 10%

Quinoa Breakfast Bowl:

Ingredients

1/2 cup cooked quinoa

1/4 cup almond milk

1 tbsp almond butter

Sliced banana and a sprinkle of cinnamon

Preparation

Mix cooked quinoa with almond milk.

Stir in almond butter and top with banana slices and cinnamon.

Nutritional Information (per serving)

Calories: 280

Protein: 8g

Fiber: 6g

Sweet Potato and Kale Hash:

Ingredients

1 medium sweet potato, grated

1 cup kale, chopped

1 tbsp olive oil

2 eggs (optional)

Preparation

Sauté sweet potato and kale in olive oil until cooked.

Top with a fried or poached egg if desired.

Nutritional Information (per serving)

Calories: 220

Protein: 7g

Vitamin A: 150%

Blueberry Almond Smoothie:

Ingredients

1 cup almond milk

1/2 cup blueberries (fresh or frozen)

1 tbsp almond butter

1 scoop protein powder (optional)

Preparation

Blend almond milk, blueberries, and almond butter until smooth.

Add protein powder if desired and blend again.

Nutritional Information (per serving)

Calories: 230

Protein: 15g

Antioxidants from blueberries

Cottage Cheese and Pineapple Bowl:

Ingredients

1/2 cup cottage cheese

1/2 cup pineapple chunks

1 tbsp flaxseeds

1 tsp honey

Preparation

Combine cottage cheese and pineapple in a bowl.

Sprinkle with flaxseeds and drizzle with honey.

Nutritional Information (per serving)

Calories: 180

Protein: 15g

Healthy Fats: 5g

Turmeric Ginger Smoothie:

Ingredients

1 cup coconut milk

1/2 tsp turmeric powder

1/2 inch ginger, grated

1/2 banana

Preparation

Blend coconut milk, turmeric, ginger, and banana until smooth.

Optionally, add ice for a refreshing twist.

Nutritional Information (per serving)

Calories: 180

Anti-inflammatory benefits from turmeric and ginger

Oatmeal with Almond Butter and Banana:

Ingredients

1/2 cup rolled oats

1 cup almond milk

1 tbsp almond butter

1/2 banana, sliced

Preparation

Cook oats in almond milk until creamy.

Stir in almond butter and top with banana slices.

Nutritional Information (per serving)

Calories: 250

Protein: 7g

Fiber: 5g

Salmon and Avocado Wrap:

Ingredients

1 whole-grain wrap

3 oz smoked salmon

1/2 avocado, sliced

Handful of spinach leaves

Preparation

Lay out the wrap and layer with smoked salmon, avocado, and spinach.

Roll the wrap and slice in half.

Nutritional Information (per serving)

Calories: 320

Protein: 20g

Omega-3 Fatty Acids from salmon

Mango and Coconut Chia Pudding:

Ingredients

2 tbsp chia seeds

1 cup coconut milk

1/2 ripe mango, diced

1 tbsp shredded coconut

Preparation

Mix chia seeds and coconut milk, refrigerate until set.

Top with diced mango and shredded coconut before serving.

Nutritional Information (per serving)

Calories: 230

Fiber: 8g

Vitamin C from mango

Egg and Veggie Breakfast Burrito:

Ingredients

2 eggs, scrambled

1 whole-grain tortilla

1/2 cup sautéed bell peppers and onions

2 tbsp salsa

Preparation

Fill the tortilla with scrambled eggs, sautéed veggies, and salsa.

Roll into a burrito and enjoy.

Nutritional Information (per serving)

Calories: 280

Protein: 14g

Fiber: 6g

Peanut Butter Banana Smoothie:

Ingredients

1 cup almond milk

1 banana

2 tbsp peanut butter

1 tbsp flaxseeds

Preparation

Blend almond milk, banana, peanut butter, and flaxseeds until smooth.

Optional: Add ice for a colder texture.

Nutritional Information (per serving)

Calories: 300

Protein: 8g

Healthy Fats: 16g

Vegetable Frittata:

Ingredients

4 eggs

1/2 cup cherry tomatoes, halved

1/2 cup baby spinach

1/4 cup feta cheese, crumbled

Preparation

Whisk eggs and pour into a greased oven-safe pan.

Add tomatoes, spinach, and feta. Bake until set.

Nutritional Information (per serving)

Calories: 240

Protein: 18g

Calcium: 15%

Almond and Berry Breakfast Quinoa:

Ingredients

1/2 cup cooked quinoa

1/4 cup almond milk

Handful of mixed berries

1 tbsp sliced almonds

Preparation

Mix cooked quinoa with almond milk.

Top with mixed berries and sliced almonds.

Nutritional Information (per serving)

Calories: 260

Protein: 7g

Antioxidants from berries

Yogurt and Berry Parfait with Nuts:

Ingredients

1 cup Greek yogurt

1/2 cup mixed berries

2 tbsp chopped nuts (almonds, walnuts)

1 tbsp honey

Preparation

Layer Greek yogurt, berries, and nuts in a glass.

Drizzle with honey before serving.

Nutritional Information (per serving)

Calories: 280

Protein: 20g

Healthy Fats: 15g

Pumpkin Spice Oatmeal:

Ingredients

1/2 cup rolled oats

1 cup almond milk

1/4 cup canned pumpkin puree

1/2 tsp pumpkin spice

Preparation

Cook oats in almond milk, stir in pumpkin puree and spice.

Optional: Top with a sprinkle of cinnamon.

Nutritional Information (per serving)

Calories: 220

Fiber: 7g

Vitamin A from pumpkin

Cranberry Walnut Overnight Oats:

Ingredients

1/2 cup rolled oats

1/2 cup Greek yogurt

1/4 cup dried cranberries

1 tbsp chopped walnuts

Preparation

Mix oats, Greek yogurt, cranberries, and walnuts in a jar.

Refrigerate overnight and stir before serving.

Nutritional Information (per serving)

Calories: 270

Protein: 13g

Omega-3 Fatty Acids from walnuts

Mushroom and Spinach Whole-Grain Toast:

Ingredients

2 slices whole-grain bread

1 cup sliced mushrooms

1 cup baby spinach

1 clove garlic, minced

Preparation

Sauté mushrooms and garlic until tender, add spinach.

Spread the mixture on toasted bread slices.

Nutritional Information (per serving)

Calories: 230

Protein: 12g

Iron from spinach

PERIMENOPAUSE DIET LUNCH RECIPES

Salmon and Quinoa Salad:

Ingredients

1 cup cooked quinoa

4 oz grilled salmon

Mixed greens (spinach, kale, arugula)

Cherry tomatoes, halved

Cucumber slices

Avocado slices

Olive oil and lemon dressing (olive oil, lemon juice, salt, and pepper)

Preparation

Cook quinoa according to package instructions.

Grill the salmon until it flakes easily with a fork.

In a large bowl, combine cooked quinoa, flaked salmon, mixed greens, cherry tomatoes, cucumber, and avocado slices.

Drizzle the olive oil and lemon dressing over the salad and toss gently to combine.

Nutritional Information (per serving)

Calories: 400

Protein: 25g

Healthy fats: 20g

Fiber: 8g

Vegetarian Stir-Fry:

Ingredients

Tofu cubes

Broccoli florets

Bell peppers (various colors), sliced

Carrots, julienned

Snap peas

Garlic, minced

Ginger, grated

Soy sauce

Sesame oil

Preparation

Press tofu to remove excess water, then stir-fry until golden brown.

Add garlic and ginger, followed by broccoli, bell peppers, carrots, and snap peas.

Drizzle with soy sauce and sesame oil, stir-frying until vegetables are tender-crisp.

Nutritional Information (per serving)

Calories: 320

Protein: 18g

Healthy fats: 15g

Fiber: 9g

Mediterranean Chickpea Salad:

Ingredients

1 can chickpeas, drained and rinsed

Cherry tomatoes, halved

Cucumber, diced

Red onion, finely chopped

Kalamata olives, sliced

Feta cheese, crumbled

Fresh parsley, chopped

Olive oil and balsamic vinegar dressing

Preparation

In a large bowl, combine chickpeas, cherry tomatoes, cucumber, red onion, olives, feta, and parsley.

Drizzle with olive oil and balsamic vinegar dressing, tossing gently to coat.

Nutritional Information (per serving)

Calories: 350

Protein: 15g

Healthy fats: 18g

Fiber: 10g

Turkey and Sweet Potato Skillet:

Ingredients

1 lb ground turkey

Sweet potatoes, diced

Red bell pepper, chopped

Spinach leaves

Garlic, minced

Paprika, cumin, salt, and pepper to taste

Preparation

In a large skillet, brown the ground turkey over medium heat.

Add diced sweet potatoes and cook until tender.

Stir in red bell pepper, spinach, and minced garlic. Season with paprika, cumin, salt, and pepper.

Nutritional Information (per serving)

Calories: 380

Protein: 28g

Healthy fats: 12g

Fiber: 7g

Quinoa and Black Bean Bowl:

Ingredients

1 cup cooked quinoa

Black beans, drained and rinsed

Corn kernels

Avocado, diced

Salsa

Lime juice

Fresh cilantro, chopped

Preparation

Cook quinoa according to package instructions.

In a bowl, combine cooked quinoa, black beans, corn, and diced avocado.

Top with salsa, a squeeze of lime juice, and fresh cilantro.

Nutritional Information (per serving)

Calories: 340

Protein: 12g

Healthy fats: 15g

Fiber: 11g

Spinach and Mushroom Quiche:

Ingredients

Pie crust (whole wheat or alternative)

Eggs

Spinach, chopped

Mushrooms, sliced

Feta cheese, crumbled

Milk (dairy or plant-based)

Salt, pepper, and nutmeg to taste

Preparation

Preheat oven and bake pie crust according to package instructions.

Sauté mushrooms and spinach until cooked.

In a bowl, whisk eggs, add milk, salt, pepper, and nutmeg. Mix in sautéed vegetables and feta.

Pour the mixture into the baked pie crust and bake until set.

Nutritional Information (per serving)

Calories: 280

Protein: 12g

Healthy fats: 15g

Fiber: 3g

Lentil and Vegetable Soup:

Ingredients

Red lentils, rinsed

Carrots, diced

Celery, chopped

Onion, finely chopped

Garlic, minced

Vegetable broth

Cumin, coriander, and turmeric

Lemon juice

Preparation

In a pot, sauté onions and garlic. Add carrots, celery, lentils, and spices.

Pour in vegetable broth, bring to a boil, then simmer until lentils and vegetables are tender.

Finish with a squeeze of lemon juice.

Nutritional Information (per serving)

Calories: 250

Protein: 18g

Healthy fats: 2g

Fiber: 12g

Chicken and Vegetable Lettuce Wraps:

Ingredients

Ground chicken

Lettuce leaves (such as iceberg or butter lettuce)

Bell peppers, thinly sliced

Carrots, julienned

Water chestnuts, chopped

Soy sauce, ginger, and garlic

Preparation

Sauté ground chicken until cooked. Add soy sauce, ginger, and garlic.

Spoon the chicken mixture into lettuce leaves.

Top with sliced bell peppers, julienned carrots, and water chestnuts.

Nutritional Information (per serving)

Calories: 320

Protein: 25g

Healthy fats: 10g

Fiber: 5g

Sweet Potato and Chickpea Curry:

Ingredients

Sweet potatoes, diced

Chickpeas, drained and rinsed

Coconut milk

Curry powder, cumin, and coriander

Onion, diced

Garlic, minced

Spinach leaves

Preparation

Sauté onions and garlic, add sweet potatoes, chickpeas, and spices.

Pour in coconut milk and simmer until sweet potatoes are tender.

Stir in spinach until wilted.

Nutritional Information (per serving)

Calories: 380

Protein: 12g

Healthy fats: 15g

Fiber: 10g

Shrimp and Avocado Wrap:

Ingredients

Whole grain wraps

Shrimp, cooked and peeled

Avocado, sliced

Cherry tomatoes, halved

Red onion, thinly sliced

Greek yogurt sauce (Greek yogurt, lime juice, cilantro)

Preparation

Lay out wraps and layer with shrimp, avocado, cherry tomatoes, and red onion.

Drizzle with Greek yogurt sauce.

Roll up and enjoy!

Nutritional Information (per serving)

Calories: 320

Protein: 20g

Healthy fats: 15g

Fiber: 8g

Cauliflower and Broccoli Quinoa Bowl:

Ingredients

Quinoa

Cauliflower florets

Broccoli florets

Chickpeas, drained and rinsed

Lemon-tahini dressing

Preparation

Roast cauliflower, broccoli, and chickpeas in the oven until golden.

Cook quinoa according to package instructions.

Assemble bowls with quinoa, roasted vegetables, and drizzle with lemon-tahini dressing.

Nutritional Information (per serving)

Calories: 340

Protein: 15g

Healthy fats: 12g

Fiber: 10g

Tofu and Vegetable Stir-Fry with Brown Rice:

Ingredients

Firm tofu, cubed

Broccoli florets

Snap peas

Carrots, thinly sliced

Brown rice, cooked

Soy sauce, ginger, and garlic

Preparation

Sauté tofu until golden. Add vegetables and stir-fry until crisp-tender.

Mix in soy sauce, ginger, and garlic.

Serve over cooked brown rice.

Nutritional Information (per serving)

Calories: 320

Protein: 18g

Healthy fats: 10g

Fiber: 8g

Turkey and Quinoa Stuffed Bell Peppers:

Ingredients

Bell peppers, halved

Ground turkey

Quinoa, cooked

Black beans, drained and rinsed

Tomato sauce

Chili powder, cumin, and garlic powder

Preparation

Preheat oven. Cook ground turkey and season with chili powder, cumin, and garlic powder.

Mix cooked quinoa, black beans, and tomato sauce.

Stuff bell peppers and bake until peppers are tender.

Nutritional Information (per serving)

Calories: 340

Protein: 25g

Healthy fats: 10g

Fiber: 10g

Salmon and Asparagus Foil Packets:

Ingredients

Salmon fillets

Asparagus spears

Lemon slices

Dill, salt, and pepper

Preparation

Preheat oven. Place salmon fillets on foil, surround with asparagus.

Season with dill, salt, and pepper. Add lemon slices.

Seal foil packets and bake until salmon is cooked through.

Nutritional Information (per serving)

Calories: 320

Protein: 25g

Healthy fats: 18g

Fiber: 5g

Caprese Quinoa Bowl:

Ingredients

Quinoa, cooked

Cherry tomatoes, halved

Fresh mozzarella, diced

Fresh basil leaves

Balsamic glaze

Preparation

Arrange quinoa in bowls, top with cherry tomatoes, mozzarella, and fresh basil.

Drizzle with balsamic glaze before serving.

Nutritional Information (per serving)

Calories: 300

Protein: 15g

Healthy fats: 15g

Fiber: 5g

Chickpea and Avocado Salad:

Ingredients

Chickpeas, drained and rinsed

Avocado, diced

Cucumber, chopped

Red onion, finely sliced

Fresh cilantro, chopped

Olive oil and lime dressing

Preparation

In a bowl, combine chickpeas, avocado, cucumber, red onion, and cilantro.

Drizzle with olive oil and lime dressing, toss gently to combine.

Nutritional Information (per serving)

Calories: 320

Protein: 12g

Healthy fats: 18g

Fiber: 10g

Mango and Shrimp Quinoa Bowl:

Ingredients

Quinoa, cooked

Shrimp, cooked and peeled

Mango, diced

Red bell pepper, chopped

Red onion, finely diced

Lime vinaigrette dressing

Preparation

Combine quinoa, shrimp, mango, bell pepper, and red onion in a bowl.

Drizzle with lime vinaigrette dressing and toss gently.

Nutritional Information (per serving)

Calories: 340

Protein: 20g

Healthy fats: 12g

Fiber: 8g

Turkey and Vegetable Skewers:

Ingredients

Turkey breast, cut into cubes

Bell peppers (various colors), cut into chunks

Zucchini, sliced

Cherry tomatoes

Olive oil, garlic, and rosemary marinade

Preparation

Marinate turkey cubes in olive oil, garlic, and rosemary.

Thread turkey, bell peppers, zucchini, and cherry tomatoes onto skewers.

Grill until turkey is cooked through and vegetables are tender.

Nutritional Information (per serving)

Calories: 280

Protein: 25g

Healthy fats: 10g

Fiber: 6g

Egg Salad Lettuce Wraps:

Ingredients

Hard-boiled eggs, chopped

Greek yogurt

Dijon mustard

Celery, finely chopped

Green onions, sliced

Lettuce leaves

Preparation

Mix chopped eggs, Greek yogurt, Dijon mustard, celery, and green onions in a bowl.

Spoon the egg salad into lettuce leaves for wraps.

Nutritional Information (per serving)

Calories: 240

Protein: 18g

Healthy fats: 15g

Fiber: 3g

Pesto Chicken and Vegetable Quinoa Bowl:

Ingredients

Chicken breast, grilled and sliced

Quinoa, cooked

Cherry tomatoes, halved

Artichoke hearts, chopped

Kalamata olives, sliced

Pesto sauce

Preparation

Assemble bowls with quinoa, grilled chicken, cherry tomatoes, artichoke hearts, and Kalamata olives.

Drizzle with pesto sauce and toss gently.

Nutritional Information (per serving)

Calories: 380

Protein: 25g

Healthy fats: 15g

Fiber: 9g

PERIMENOPAUSE DIET DINNER RECIPES

Grilled Salmon with Avocado Salsa

Ingredients

Salmon fillets

Olive oil

Salt and pepper

Avocado

Tomato

Red onion

Cilantro

Lime juice

Preparation

Season salmon with salt, pepper, and olive oil.

Grill salmon until cooked.

Mix diced avocado, tomato, red onion, cilantro, and lime juice for salsa.

Serve salmon with avocado salsa.

Nutritional Information (per serving)

Calories: 350

Protein: 25g

Healthy fats: 20g

Carbohydrates: 15g

Quinoa and Vegetable Stir-Fry

Ingredients

Quinoa

Mixed vegetables (bell peppers, broccoli, carrots, snap peas)

Tofu or chicken

Soy sauce

Garlic

Ginger

Sesame oil

Preparation

Cook quinoa according to package instructions.

Stir-fry tofu/chicken with vegetables, garlic, and ginger in sesame oil.

Add cooked quinoa and soy sauce, stir until combined.

Nutritional Information (per serving)

Calories: 400

Protein: 18g

Healthy fats: 15g

Carbohydrates: 45g

Spinach and Mushroom Stuffed Chicken Breast

Ingredients

Chicken breasts

Spinach

Mushrooms

Feta cheese

Olive oil

Garlic

Lemon juice

Thyme

Preparation

Sauté spinach, mushrooms, garlic, and thyme in olive oil.

Cut a pocket in each chicken breast and stuff with the sautéed mixture.

Bake until chicken is cooked, then sprinkle with feta and lemon juice.

Nutritional Information (per serving)

Calories: 320

Protein: 35g

Healthy fats: 15g

Carbohydrates: 10g

Lentil and Vegetable Curry

Ingredients

Lentils

Cauliflower

Carrots

Bell peppers

Coconut milk

Curry powder

Turmeric

Cumin

Coriander

Preparation

Cook lentils as per package instructions.

Sauté vegetables in curry powder, turmeric, cumin, and coriander.

Add cooked lentils and coconut milk, simmer until vegetables are tender.

Nutritional Information (per serving)

Calories: 300

Protein: 15g

Healthy fats: 10g

Carbohydrates: 40g

Sweet Potato and Chickpea Buddha Bowl

Ingredients

Sweet potatoes

Chickpeas

Quinoa

Kale

Avocado

Tahini

Lemon juice

Olive oil

Preparation

Roast sweet potatoes and chickpeas with olive oil and spices.

Cook quinoa and massage kale with olive oil.

Assemble bowls with roasted veggies, quinoa, kale, and sliced avocado. Drizzle with tahini and lemon juice.

Nutritional Information (per serving)

Calories: 380

Protein: 15g

Healthy fats: 18g

Carbohydrates: 45g

Turkey and Vegetable Skewers

Ingredients

Turkey breast

Zucchini

Cherry tomatoes

Red onion

Olive oil

Lemon juice

Oregano

Garlic

Preparation

Cut turkey into cubes and marinate in olive oil, lemon juice, oregano, and garlic.

Skewer turkey, zucchini, cherry tomatoes, and red onion.

Grill until turkey is cooked and vegetables are charred.

Nutritional Information (per serving)

Calories: 280

Protein: 30g

Healthy fats: 12g

Carbohydrates: 15g

Cauliflower Fried Rice

Ingredients

Cauliflower rice

Shrimp or tofu

Mixed vegetables (peas, carrots, corn)

Egg

Soy sauce

Sesame oil

Green onions

Preparation

Sauté shrimp/tofu, vegetables, and cauliflower rice in sesame oil.

Push ingredients to the side, scramble egg in the pan.

Mix everything together, add soy sauce, and garnish with green onions.

Nutritional Information (per serving)

Calories: 250

Protein: 20g

Healthy fats: 10g

Carbohydrates: 25g

Mediterranean Stuffed Bell Peppers

Ingredients

Bell peppers

Ground turkey or chicken

Quinoa

Spinach

Feta cheese

Cherry tomatoes

Kalamata olives

Olive oil

Oregano

Preparation

Cook quinoa and brown ground turkey/chicken.

Mix quinoa, turkey/chicken, spinach, feta, tomatoes, olives, olive oil, and oregano.

Stuff bell peppers with the mixture and bake until peppers are tender.

Nutritional Information (per serving)

Calories: 320

Protein: 25g

Healthy fats: 15g

Carbohydrates: 25g

Broccoli and Chicken Stir-Fry with Cashews

Ingredients

Chicken breasts

Broccoli

Cashews

Soy sauce

Hoisin sauce

Ginger

Garlic

Sesame oil

Preparation

Stir-fry chicken, broccoli, ginger, and garlic in sesame oil.

Add soy sauce and hoisin sauce, cook until chicken is done.

Top with cashews before serving.

Nutritional Information (per serving)

Calories: 350

Protein: 30g

Healthy fats: 18g

Carbohydrates: 20g

Greek Salad with Grilled Chicken

Ingredients

Chicken breasts

Romaine lettuce

Cucumber

Cherry tomatoes

Red onion

Feta cheese

Kalamata olives

Olive oil

Lemon juice

Oregano

Preparation

Grill chicken until cooked.

Combine lettuce, cucumber, tomatoes, red onion, feta, and olives.

Top with grilled chicken and dress with olive oil, lemon juice, and oregano.

Nutritional Information (per serving)

Calories: 320

Protein: 30g

Healthy fats: 15g

Carbohydrates: 15g

Salmon and Asparagus Foil Packets

Ingredients

Salmon fillets

Asparagus spears

Lemon slices

Garlic

Dill

Olive oil

Salt and pepper

Preparation

Place salmon on a foil sheet, surround with asparagus.

Drizzle with olive oil, add minced garlic, dill, salt, and pepper.

Seal foil packets and bake until salmon is cooked.

Nutritional Information (per serving)

Calories: 300

Protein: 30g

Healthy fats: 18g

Carbohydrates: 8g

Turkey and Sweet Potato Chili

Ingredients

Ground turkey

Sweet potatoes

Black beans

Diced tomatoes

Chili powder

Cumin

Paprika

Onion

Garlic

Chicken broth

Preparation

Brown turkey with onions and garlic.

Add sweet potatoes, black beans, diced tomatoes, spices, and chicken broth.

Simmer until sweet potatoes are tender.

Nutritional Information (per serving)

Calories: 350

Protein: 25g

Healthy fats: 10g

Carbohydrates: 40g

Cauliflower and Broccoli Gratin

Ingredients

Cauliflower florets

Broccoli florets

Cheddar cheese

Greek yogurt

Dijon mustard

Garlic powder

Salt and pepper

Breadcrumbs (optional)

Preparation

Steam cauliflower and broccoli until tender.

Mix Greek yogurt, Dijon mustard, garlic powder, salt, and pepper.

Combine veggies with the yogurt mixture, top with cheese (and breadcrumbs if desired), and bake until bubbly.

Nutritional Information (per serving)

Calories: 280

Protein: 15g

Healthy fats: 12g

Carbohydrates: 30g

Shrimp and Vegetable Stir-Fry with Brown Rice

Ingredients

Shrimp

Broccoli

Bell peppers

Snap peas

Carrots

Soy sauce

Ginger

Garlic

Brown rice

Preparation

Stir-fry shrimp and veggies in soy sauce, ginger, and garlic.

Serve over cooked brown rice.

Nutritional Information (per serving)

Calories: 320

Protein: 20g

Healthy fats: 8g

Carbohydrates: 45g

Mushroom and Spinach Stuffed Portobello Mushrooms

Ingredients

Portobello mushrooms

Spinach

Mushrooms

Feta cheese

Olive oil

Balsamic vinegar

Garlic

Thyme

Preparation

Remove mushroom stems, sauté with spinach, mushrooms, garlic, and thyme in olive oil.

Stuff portobello caps with the mixture, top with feta.

Drizzle with balsamic vinegar and bake until mushrooms are tender.

Nutritional Information (per serving)

Calories: 220

Protein: 15g

Healthy fats: 12g

Carbohydrates: 18g

Chicken and Vegetable Skillet with Quinoa

Ingredients

Chicken thighs

Quinoa

Bell peppers

Zucchini

Cherry tomatoes

Onion

Garlic

Chicken broth

Italian seasoning

Preparation

Sear chicken in a skillet, remove.

Sauté veggies and garlic, add quinoa, chicken broth, and Italian seasoning.

Place chicken on top, cover, and simmer until quinoa is cooked.

Nutritional Information (per serving)

Calories: 380

Protein: 25g

Healthy fats: 15g

Carbohydrates: 35g

Lemon Herb Baked Cod

Ingredients

Cod fillets

Lemon juice

Olive oil

Garlic

Parsley

Dill

Salt and pepper

Preparation

Marinate cod in lemon juice, olive oil, minced garlic, parsley, dill, salt, and pepper.

Bake until fish is opaque and flakes easily.

Nutritional Information (per serving)

Calories: 250

Protein: 30g

Healthy fats: 12g

Carbohydrates: 2g

Eggplant and Chickpea Curry

Ingredients

Eggplant

Chickpeas

Coconut milk

Curry powder

Cumin

Coriander

Turmeric

Ginger

Garlic

Basmati rice

Preparation

Sauté eggplant, chickpeas, ginger, and garlic in curry powder, cumin, coriander, and turmeric.

Add coconut milk, simmer until eggplant is tender.

Serve over cooked basmati rice.

Nutritional Information (per serving)

Calories: 320

Protein: 10g

Healthy fats: 15g

Carbohydrates: 40g

Pesto Zoodles with Grilled Chicken

Ingredients

Zucchini noodles (zoodles)

Grilled chicken breast

Cherry tomatoes

Pesto sauce

Parmesan cheese

Pine nuts

Preparation

Sauté zoodles and cherry tomatoes in pesto sauce.

Top with grilled chicken, Parmesan, and pine nuts.

Nutritional Information (per serving)

Calories: 300

Protein: 25g

Healthy fats: 18g

Carbohydrates: 12g

Beef and Vegetable Lettuce Wraps

Ingredients

Ground beef

Lettuce leaves

Bell peppers

Water chestnuts

Soy sauce

Hoisin sauce

Ginger

Garlic

Green onions

Preparation

Brown beef, add diced bell peppers, water chestnuts, ginger, and garlic.

Stir in soy sauce and hoisin sauce.

Spoon mixture into lettuce leaves, garnish with green onions.

Nutritional Information (per serving)

Calories: 280

Protein: 20g

Healthy fats: 15g

Carbohydrates: 15g

PERIMENOPAUSE DIET SOUP AND STEW RECIPES

Vegetable and Quinoa Stew

Ingredients

1 cup quinoa

4 cups vegetable broth

1 onion, chopped

2 carrots, sliced

2 zucchini, diced

1 can (15 oz) diced tomatoes

1 teaspoon dried thyme

Salt and pepper to taste

Preparation

Rinse quinoa under cold water.

In a large pot, combine quinoa, vegetable broth, onion, carrots, zucchini, tomatoes, thyme, salt, and pepper.

Bring to a boil, then reduce heat and simmer for 20-25 minutes or until quinoa and vegetables are tender.

Nutritional Information

Serving Size: 1.5 cups

Calories: 220

Protein: 8g

Fiber: 6g

Chicken and Wild Rice Soup

Ingredients

1 cup wild rice

4 cups chicken broth

1 lb boneless, skinless chicken breast, cooked and shredded

1 cup celery, chopped

1 cup carrots, sliced

1 onion, diced

2 cloves garlic, minced

1 teaspoon dried thyme

Salt and pepper to taste

Preparation

Cook wild rice according to package instructions.

In a large pot, combine chicken broth, cooked chicken, celery, carrots, onion, garlic, thyme, salt, and pepper.

Simmer for 15-20 minutes or until vegetables are tender.

Nutritional Information

Serving Size: 1.5 cups

Calories: 280

Protein: 22g

Fiber: 4g

Lentil and Spinach Soup

Ingredients

1 cup dried green lentils, rinsed

6 cups vegetable broth

1 onion, chopped

2 carrots, diced

3 cloves garlic, minced

1 teaspoon ground cumin

1 teaspoon paprika

4 cups fresh spinach

Preparation

In a large pot, combine lentils, vegetable broth, onion, carrots, garlic, cumin, and paprika.

Bring to a boil, then reduce heat and simmer for 25-30 minutes or until lentils are tender.

Add spinach and cook until wilted.

Nutritional Information

Serving Size: 1.5 cups

Calories: 240

Protein: 16g

Fiber: 12g

Salmon and Sweet Potato Chowder

Ingredients

1 lb salmon fillet, cut into chunks

2 sweet potatoes, peeled and diced

1 onion, finely chopped

2 celery stalks, diced

2 cups corn kernels

4 cups vegetable broth

1 cup milk or unsweetened almond milk

1 teaspoon dill

Salt and pepper to taste

Preparation

In a large pot, combine salmon, sweet potatoes, onion, celery, corn, vegetable broth, milk, dill, salt, and pepper.

Simmer for 20-25 minutes or until sweet potatoes are tender.

Nutritional Information

Serving Size: 1.5 cups

Calories: 300

Protein: 22g

Fiber: 5g

Mushroom and Barley Soup

Ingredients

1 cup pearl barley

8 cups vegetable broth

1 lb mushrooms, sliced

1 onion, chopped

3 carrots, diced

3 celery stalks, chopped

2 cloves garlic, minced

1 teaspoon dried thyme

Salt and pepper to taste

Preparation

Rinse barley under cold water.

In a large pot, combine barley, vegetable broth, mushrooms, onion, carrots, celery, garlic, thyme, salt, and pepper.

Simmer for 30-35 minutes or until barley is tender.

Nutritional Information

Serving Size: 1.5 cups

Calories: 230

Protein: 8g

Fiber: 10g

Tomato and Chickpea Soup

Ingredients

2 cans (15 oz each) chickpeas, drained and rinsed

1 onion, diced

3 cloves garlic, minced

1 can (28 oz) crushed tomatoes

4 cups vegetable broth

1 teaspoon dried oregano

1 teaspoon dried basil

Salt and pepper to taste

Preparation

In a large pot, combine chickpeas, onion, garlic, crushed tomatoes, vegetable broth, oregano, basil, salt, and pepper.

Bring to a boil, then reduce heat and simmer for 15-20 minutes.

Nutritional Information

Serving Size: 1.5 cups

Calories: 220

Protein: 10g

Fiber: 8g

Turkey and Vegetable Chili

Ingredients

1 lb ground turkey

1 onion, chopped

3 cloves garlic, minced

1 bell pepper, diced

2 cans (15 oz each) black beans, drained and rinsed

1 can (28 oz) diced tomatoes

1 cup frozen corn

2 teaspoons chili powder

1 teaspoon cumin

Salt and pepper to taste

Preparation

In a large pot, cook ground turkey until browned.

Add onion, garlic, bell pepper, black beans, diced tomatoes, corn, chili powder, cumin, salt, and pepper.

Simmer for 20-25 minutes.

Nutritional Information

Serving Size: 1.5 cups

Calories: 280

Protein: 20g

Fiber: 9g

Butternut Squash and Apple Soup

Ingredients

1 medium butternut squash, peeled and diced

2 apples, peeled and chopped

1 onion, chopped

4 cups vegetable broth

1 teaspoon curry powder

1/2 teaspoon cinnamon

Salt and pepper to taste

Preparation

In a large pot, combine butternut squash, apples, onion, vegetable broth, curry powder, cinnamon, salt, and pepper.

Simmer for 20-25 minutes or until squash and apples are tender.

Blend until smooth.

Nutritional Information

Serving Size: 1.5 cups

Calories: 180

Protein: 2g

Fiber: 6g

Spinach and White Bean Stew

Ingredients

2 cans (15 oz each) white beans, drained and rinsed

1 onion, diced

3 cloves garlic, minced

1 can (14 oz) diced tomatoes

4 cups vegetable broth

4 cups fresh spinach

1 teaspoon dried rosemary

Salt and pepper to taste

Preparation

In a large pot, combine white beans, onion, garlic, diced tomatoes, vegetable broth, spinach, rosemary, salt, and pepper.

Simmer for 15-20 minutes or until spinach is wilted.

Nutritional Information

Serving Size: 1.5 cups

Calories: 200

Protein: 10g

Fiber: 8g

Shrimp and Vegetable Gumbo

Ingredients

1 lb shrimp, peeled and deveined

1 onion, chopped

1 bell pepper, diced

3 celery stalks, chopped

2 cloves garlic, minced

1 can (14 oz) diced tomatoes

4 cups vegetable broth

1 teaspoon Cajun seasoning

1/2 teaspoon dried thyme

Salt and pepper to taste

Preparation

In a large pot, cook shrimp until pink. Remove and set aside.

In the same pot, sauté onion, bell pepper, celery, and garlic until softened.

Add diced tomatoes, vegetable broth, Cajun seasoning, thyme, salt, and pepper. Bring to a boil, then simmer for 15-20 minutes.

Add cooked shrimp back to the pot and heat through.

Nutritional Information

Serving Size: 1.5 cups

Calories: 220

Protein: 25g

Fiber: 5g

Sweet Potato and Kale Soup

Ingredients

2 large sweet potatoes, peeled and diced

1 bunch kale, stems removed and leaves chopped

1 onion, finely chopped

3 cloves garlic, minced

4 cups vegetable broth

1 can (14 oz) coconut milk

1 teaspoon turmeric

Salt and pepper to taste

Preparation

In a large pot, combine sweet potatoes, kale, onion, garlic, vegetable broth, coconut milk, turmeric, salt, and pepper.

Simmer for 20-25 minutes or until sweet potatoes are tender.

Nutritional Information

Serving Size: 1.5 cups

Calories: 250

Protein: 5g

Fiber: 8g

Broccoli and Cheddar Soup

Ingredients

2 cups broccoli florets

1 onion, chopped

2 carrots, diced

3 cups vegetable broth

2 cups shredded cheddar cheese

1 cup milk or unsweetened almond milk

2 tablespoons whole wheat flour

Salt and pepper to taste

Preparation

In a large pot, combine broccoli, onion, carrots, vegetable broth, cheddar cheese, milk, flour, salt, and pepper.

Simmer for 15-20 minutes or until vegetables are tender.

Nutritional Information

Serving Size: 1.5 cups

Calories: 320

Protein: 15g

Fiber: 4g

Cauliflower and Leek Soup

Ingredients

1 head cauliflower, chopped

2 leeks, sliced

3 cloves garlic, minced

4 cups vegetable broth

1 cup unsweetened almond milk

1 teaspoon thyme

1/2 teaspoon nutmeg

Salt and pepper to taste

Preparation

In a large pot, combine cauliflower, leeks, garlic, vegetable broth, almond milk, thyme, nutmeg, salt, and pepper.

Simmer for 20-25 minutes or until cauliflower is tender.

Nutritional Information

Serving Size: 1.5 cups

Calories: 180

Protein: 5g

Fiber: 8g

Turkey and Quinoa Chili

Ingredients

1 lb ground turkey

1 onion, diced

3 cloves garlic, minced

1 bell pepper, chopped

1 can (15 oz) black beans, drained and rinsed

1 can (14 oz) diced tomatoes

1 cup cooked quinoa

2 teaspoons chili powder

1 teaspoon cumin

Salt and pepper to taste

Preparation

In a large pot, cook ground turkey until browned.

Add onion, garlic, bell pepper, black beans, diced tomatoes, cooked quinoa, chili powder, cumin, salt, and pepper.

Simmer for 20-25 minutes.

Nutritional Information

Serving Size: 1.5 cups

Calories: 290

Protein: 22g

Fiber: 9g

Spaghetti Squash and Meatball Soup

Ingredients

1 medium spaghetti squash, cooked and shredded

1 lb lean ground beef or turkey

1 onion, finely chopped

2 carrots, diced

2 cloves garlic, minced

1 can (14 oz) crushed tomatoes

4 cups beef or vegetable broth

1 teaspoon Italian seasoning

Salt and pepper to taste

Preparation

In a large pot, cook ground beef or turkey until browned.

Add onion, carrots, garlic, crushed tomatoes, shredded spaghetti squash, broth, Italian seasoning, salt, and pepper.

Simmer for 15-20 minutes.

Nutritional Information

Serving Size: 1.5 cups

Calories: 260

Protein: 22g

Fiber: 7g

Red Lentil and Vegetable Curry Soup

Ingredients

1 cup red lentils, rinsed

1 onion, chopped

2 carrots, sliced

1 zucchini, diced

3 cups vegetable broth

1 can (14 oz) coconut milk

2 tablespoons red curry paste

1 teaspoon turmeric

Salt and pepper to taste

Preparation

In a large pot, combine red lentils, onion, carrots, zucchini, vegetable broth, coconut milk, red curry paste, turmeric, salt, and pepper.

Bring to a boil, then reduce heat and simmer for 20-25 minutes or until lentils are tender.

Nutritional Information

Serving Size: 1.5 cups

Calories: 280

Protein: 14g

Fiber: 8g

Mexican Chicken and Quinoa Soup

Ingredients

1 lb chicken breasts, cooked and shredded

1 onion, diced

1 bell pepper, chopped

1 can (15 oz) black beans, drained and rinsed

1 cup corn kernels

1 cup cooked quinoa

4 cups chicken broth

1 can (14 oz) diced tomatoes with green chilies

1 teaspoon cumin

Salt and pepper to taste

Preparation

In a large pot, combine shredded chicken, onion, bell pepper, black beans, corn, quinoa, chicken broth, diced tomatoes, cumin, salt, and pepper.

Simmer for 15-20 minutes.

Nutritional Information

Serving Size: 1.5 cups

Calories: 290

Protein: 28g

Fiber: 8g

Miso and Vegetable Noodle Soup

Ingredients

6 cups vegetable broth

3 tablespoons miso paste

1 cup shiitake mushrooms, sliced

1 cup bok choy, chopped

1 carrot, julienned

2 green onions, sliced

2 cups cooked soba noodles

1 tablespoon soy sauce

1 teaspoon sesame oil

Preparation

In a large pot, whisk miso paste into vegetable broth until dissolved.

Add shiitake mushrooms, bok choy, carrot, green onions, soba noodles, soy sauce, and sesame oil.

Simmer for 10-15 minutes.

Nutritional Information

Serving Size: 1.5 cups

Calories: 180

Protein: 8g

Fiber: 4g

Black-Eyed Pea and Collard Green Soup

Ingredients

2 cans (15 oz each) black-eyed peas, drained and rinsed

1 bunch collard greens, stems removed and leaves chopped

1 onion, chopped

2 carrots, diced

3 cloves garlic, minced

4 cups vegetable broth

1 teaspoon smoked paprika

Salt and pepper to taste

Preparation

In a large pot, combine black-eyed peas, collard greens, onion, carrots, garlic, vegetable broth, smoked paprika, salt, and pepper.

Simmer for 20-25 minutes.

Nutritional Information

Serving Size: 1.5 cups

Calories: 210

Protein: 10g

Fiber: 9g

Quinoa and Kale Minestrone

Ingredients

1 cup quinoa, rinsed

1 bunch kale, stems removed and leaves chopped

2 carrots, sliced

1 zucchini, diced

1 can (15 oz) kidney beans, drained and rinsed

1 can (14 oz) diced tomatoes

4 cups vegetable broth

1 teaspoon Italian seasoning

Salt and pepper to taste

Preparation

In a large pot, combine quinoa, kale, carrots, zucchini, kidney beans, diced tomatoes, vegetable broth, Italian seasoning, salt, and pepper.

Simmer for 20-25 minutes or until quinoa is cooked.

Nutritional Information

Serving Size: 1.5 cups

Calories: 240

Protein: 10g

Fiber: 8g

PERIMENOPAUSE DIET SALAD RECIPES

Superfood Spinach Salad:

Ingredients

Fresh spinach leaves

Quinoa (cooked)

Cherry tomatoes

Avocado (sliced)

Walnuts (chopped)

Feta cheese (crumbled)

Dressing:

Olive oil

Lemon juice

Dijon mustard

Salt and pepper to taste

Preparation

Toss all salad ingredients, mix dressing separately, and drizzle over the salad.

Nutritional Information (per serving)

Calories: 300, Protein: 10g, Fiber: 8g.

Citrus Kale Salad:

Ingredients

Kale leaves (chopped)

Oranges (peeled and segmented)

Red onion (thinly sliced)

Pomegranate seeds

Pumpkin seeds

Dressing:

Olive oil

Orange juice

Honey

Salt and pepper to taste

Preparation

Massage kale with dressing, add other ingredients, and toss.

Nutritional Information (per serving)

Calories: 250, Protein: 7g, Fiber: 10g.

Mango Avocado Quinoa Salad:

Ingredients

Cooked quinoa

Mango (diced)

Avocado (diced)

Cucumber (sliced)

Red bell pepper (chopped)

Dressing:

Lime juice

Olive oil

Cilantro (chopped)

Salt and pepper to taste

Preparation

Combine salad ingredients, mix dressing, and gently toss.

Nutritional Information (per serving)

Calories: 280, Protein: 6g, Fiber: 9g.

Greek Chickpea Salad:

Ingredients

Chickpeas (canned, drained)

Cherry tomatoes (halved)

Cucumber (diced)

Kalamata olives

Red onion (chopped)

Feta cheese (crumbled)

Dressing:

Olive oil

Red wine vinegar

Garlic (minced)

Oregano (dried)

Salt and pepper to taste

Preparation

Mix salad ingredients, whisk dressing, and combine.

Nutritional Information (per serving)

Calories: 320, Protein: 11g, Fiber: 8g.

Protein-Packed Tuna Salad:

Ingredients

Mixed greens

Canned tuna (in water, drained)

Cherry tomatoes

Hard-boiled eggs (sliced)

Green beans (blanched)

Dressing:

Yogurt

Dijon mustard

Lemon juice

Salt and pepper to taste

Preparation

Arrange salad ingredients, mix dressing, and drizzle over the top.

Nutritional Information (per serving)

Calories: 290, Protein: 20g, Fiber: 6g.

Quinoa and Black Bean Fiesta Salad:

Ingredients

Cooked quinoa

Black beans (canned, rinsed)

Corn kernels (fresh or frozen)

Red bell pepper (diced)

Green onions (chopped)

Dressing:

Lime juice

Olive oil

Cumin powder

Chili powder

Salt and pepper to taste

Preparation

Combine salad ingredients, whisk dressing, and toss.

Nutritional Information (per serving)

Calories: 270, Protein: 10g, Fiber: 8g.

Cranberry Walnut Chicken Salad:

Ingredients

Grilled chicken (sliced)

Mixed greens

Dried cranberries

Walnuts (chopped)

Feta cheese (crumbled)

Dressing:

Balsamic vinegar

Olive oil

Dijon mustard

Honey

Salt and pepper to taste

Preparation

Assemble salad ingredients, mix dressing, and drizzle over the salad.

Nutritional Information (per serving)

Calories: 320, Protein: 18g, Fiber: 7g.

Roasted Vegetable Quinoa Salad:

Ingredients

Roasted vegetables (e.g., sweet potatoes, Brussels sprouts, carrots)

Cooked quinoa

Baby spinach

Pecans (toasted)

Goat cheese (crumbled)

Dressing:

Balsamic vinegar

Olive oil

Dijon mustard

Maple syrup

Salt and pepper to taste

Preparation

Combine salad ingredients, whisk dressing, and toss.

Nutritional Information (per serving)

Calories: 280, Protein: 9g, Fiber: 10g.

Caprese Salad with Basil Pesto:

Ingredients

Tomatoes (sliced)

Fresh mozzarella (sliced)

Fresh basil leaves

Pine nuts (toasted)

Pesto:

Fresh basil

Pine nuts

Garlic

Parmesan cheese

Olive oil

Preparation

Arrange tomatoes and mozzarella, top with pesto, and garnish with basil and pine nuts.

Nutritional Information (per serving)

Calories: 250, Protein: 12g, Fiber: 3g.

Asian Sesame Ginger Chicken Salad:

Ingredients

Grilled chicken (shredded)

Napa cabbage (shredded)

Carrots (julienne)

Edamame (cooked)

Mandarin oranges

Dressing:

Sesame oil

Soy sauce

Rice vinegar

Ginger (grated)

Honey

Preparation

Mix salad ingredients, whisk dressing, and toss.

Nutritional Information (per serving)

Calories: 310, Protein: 18g, Fiber: 6g.

Blueberry Almond Quinoa Salad:

Ingredients

Cooked quinoa

Blueberries

Sliced almonds (toasted)

Feta cheese (crumbled)

Cucumber (diced)

Dressing:

Lemon juice

Olive oil

Honey

Dijon mustard

Salt and pepper to taste

Preparation

Combine salad ingredients, whisk dressing, and gently toss.

Nutritional Information (per serving)

Calories: 280, Protein: 9g, Fiber: 7g.

Southwest Blackened Salmon Salad:

Ingredients

Blackened salmon fillets

Romaine lettuce

Black beans (canned, rinsed)

Corn kernels (grilled or roasted)

Cherry tomatoes

Dressing:

Greek yogurt

Lime juice

Chipotle powder

Cilantro (chopped)

Salt and pepper to taste

Preparation

Arrange salad ingredients, mix dressing, and drizzle over the top.

Nutritional Information (per serving)

Calories: 330, Protein: 25g, Fiber: 8g.

Pear and Gorgonzola Arugula Salad:

Ingredients

Arugula

Pears (sliced)

Gorgonzola cheese (crumbled)

Candied pecans

Red onion (thinly sliced)

Dressing:

Balsamic vinegar

Olive oil

Dijon mustard

Maple syrup

Salt and pepper to taste

Preparation

Toss salad ingredients, whisk dressing, and drizzle over the salad.

Nutritional Information (per serving)

Calories: 290, Protein: 7g, Fiber: 6g.

Mediterranean Chickpea and Artichoke Salad:

Ingredients

Chickpeas (canned, drained)

Artichoke hearts (canned, quartered)

Cherry tomatoes

Kalamata olives

Red onion (chopped)

Dressing:

Lemon juice

Olive oil

Garlic (minced)

Oregano (dried)

Salt and pepper to taste

Preparation

Mix salad ingredients, whisk dressing, and combine.

Nutritional Information (per serving)

Calories: 270, Protein: 9g, Fiber: 8g.

Shrimp and Avocado Salad:

Ingredients

Cooked shrimp (peeled and deveined)

Mixed greens

Avocado (sliced)

Grapefruit segments

Red onion (thinly sliced)

Dressing:

Lime juice

Olive oil

Cilantro (chopped)

Salt and pepper to taste

Preparation

Arrange salad ingredients, mix dressing, and drizzle over the top.

Nutritional Information (per serving)

Calories: 280, Protein: 20g, Fiber: 7g.

Beet and Goat Cheese Salad:

Ingredients

Roasted beets (sliced)

Mixed greens

Goat cheese (crumbled)

Walnuts (chopped)

Red onion (thinly sliced)

Dressing:

Balsamic vinegar

Olive oil

Dijon mustard

Honey

Salt and pepper to taste

Preparation

Toss salad ingredients, whisk dressing, and drizzle over the salad.

Nutritional Information (per serving)

Calories: 260, Protein: 8g, Fiber: 6g.

Cauliflower and Broccoli Detox Salad:

Ingredients

Cauliflower florets (raw)

Broccoli florets (raw)

Carrots (shredded)

Sunflower seeds

Cranberries (dried)

Dressing:

Greek yogurt

Apple cider vinegar

Honey

Poppy seeds

Salt and pepper to taste

Preparation

Combine salad ingredients, whisk dressing, and toss.

Nutritional Information (per serving)

Calories: 240, Protein: 6g, Fiber: 8g.

Tofu and Edamame Sesame Salad:

Ingredients

Firm tofu (cubed)

Edamame (cooked)

Napa cabbage (shredded)

Red bell pepper (thinly sliced)

Sesame seeds (toasted)

Dressing:

Soy sauce

Rice vinegar

Sesame oil

Ginger (grated)

Garlic (minced)

Preparation

Mix salad ingredients, whisk dressing, and gently toss.

Nutritional Information (per serving)

Calories: 250, Protein: 15g, Fiber: 7g.

Cherry Tomato and Mozzarella Salad:

Ingredients

Cherry tomatoes

Fresh mozzarella balls

Fresh basil leaves

Balsamic glaze

Olive oil

Preparation

Arrange tomatoes, mozzarella, and basil on a plate. Drizzle with olive oil and balsamic glaze.

Nutritional Information (per serving)

Calories: 220, Protein: 10g, Fiber: 3g.

Spring Asparagus and Egg Salad:

Ingredients

Asparagus (blanched and sliced)

Hard-boiled eggs (sliced)

Mixed greens

Radishes (thinly sliced)

Lemon zest

Dressing:

Dijon mustard

Olive oil

Lemon juice

Honey

Salt and pepper to taste

Preparation

Arrange salad ingredients, mix dressing, and drizzle over the top.

Nutritional Information (per serving)

Calories: 230, Protein: 12g, Fiber: 6g.

During perimenopause, women go through a profound and individual process of accepting and embracing the aging and changing that comes with this time in their lives. Having a growth mindset means keeping an open mind, embracing change, and appreciating the maturity that comes with age.

Changes in skin elasticity, metabolism, and weight gain/loss are only few of the physical manifestations of perimenopause. Accepting these shifts calls for self-love and a rethinking of beauty standards set by others. Understanding and accepting that aging is a normal aspect of life requires an appreciation for the body's resiliency.

about a psychological level, perimenopause might provoke musings about identity and purpose. As women's ability to have children changes, they may have to answer new issues about their place in society. Accepting this change means realizing that life is an ever-evolving adventure with different stages offering their own set of challenges and rewards.

Maintaining an optimistic outlook is crucial. It's about seeing becoming older not as a setback but as an opportunity to develop wisdom, fortitude, and perspective. Approaching perimenopause with an attitude of self-acceptance increases emotional well-being and resilience in the face of society demands or perceived standards.

Having a strong social network is essential for adjusting to the changes that come with perimenopause. Communicating with others about your thoughts and struggles might help you feel less alone. Talking about becoming older and making changes can help people connect with one another and give them a sense of agency.

Positive attitudes toward aging are aided by participating in pursuits that offer happiness and satisfaction. During this time of change, the sense of purpose and happiness can be bolstered by the pursuit of hobbies, the acquisition of new skills, or participation in physical activities.

A comprehensive perspective is necessary for accepting age and change during perimenopause. It's about taking care of yourself physically, mentally, and spiritually, enjoying the ride, and acknowledging that each new year has its own special set of challenges and rewards. Women may face the challenges of perimenopause with dignity, strength, and confidence if they learn to appreciate the natural elegance of the aging process.

Why You Should Not Worry

Cultivating positive thoughts on aging is a transforming mentality that transcends cultural narratives and appreciates the richness that comes with the passage of time. Viewing aging as a good and powerful experience includes redefining cultural assumptions and recognizing the unique features that each life stage provides.

To have a good outlook on becoming older, it's important to value the years of experience and knowledge that have been amassed. Every line and strand of gray hair is a testament to the person's fortitude, maturity, and adaptability over the years. Accepting these outward signs as evidence of a life well-lived might help one develop a more optimistic and grateful perspective.

One of the benefits of becoming older is the chance to become closer to one's own identity. Self-knowledge and acceptance can improve with the development of new priorities and viewpoints. Through overcoming adversity, one develops a stronger character and a more refined capacity to handle life's complications.

As we become older, it becomes even more important to cultivate deep relationships with those around us. Appreciating the rich tapestry of people at all ages and phases of life is important to a positive view of aging, as is nurturing existing relationships and making new ones. Participating in friendships, families, and other social groups all help to foster a feeling of community and common ground.

A good outlook on aging requires taking care of oneself and being healthy. Incorporating good habits, maintaining an active lifestyle, and giving attention to one's mental health all lead to increased vitality and happiness. Taking measures like scheduling frequent checkups and prioritizing self-care demonstrates a will to age positively and proactively.

Having a good outlook on becoming older is all about living in the now and looking forward to the future. Accepting oneself as one is requires letting go of judgment from others, appreciating one's own uniqueness, and seeing the beauty in the inevitable passage of time. People may age with dignity, poise, and a deep appreciation for life's ever-changing tapestry if they cultivate an optimistic outlook.

Living With Perimenopause

In order to successfully go through the many phases of life, it is essential to be open to and even seek out change and development. Rather of opposing or dreading change, engaging it with openness and a positive outlook may lead to personal growth, resilience, and a greater understanding of oneself.

One key factor in embracing change during perimenopause is acknowledging the bodily shifts that occur. Fluctuations in hormone levels, changes in skin texture, and metabolic shifts are all possible causes. To accept these alterations, one must learn to be kind to oneself and see the value in the ever-evolving person. The emphasis moves from external, normative standards to one's own strengths and values.

Perimenopause can cause a reevaluation of one's values, relationships, and life objectives on a psychological level. In this sense, accepting change is letting go of preconceived notions of who you "should" be and instead welcoming the opportunity to create a brand-new you. It's a chance for people to learn more about themselves and their place in the world.

Adapting to new circumstances may help you develop as a person and in your career. Being open to change in the job might include taking on new responsibilities, learning new abilities, or reevaluating professional aspirations. By viewing transition as an opportunity for growth, a woman in perimenopause may take charge of her professional life and flourish during this time.

Accepting change requires an optimistic outlook, which may be developed through practice. This entails rethinking difficulties as educational challenges and viewing changes as inevitable features of living. Strengthening one's capacity to bounce back from adversity gives one more agency over their own story and increases their flexibility.

When adapting to a new situation, social connections may be really helpful. Connecting with individuals who share similar experiences or seeking help from mentors and friends builds a supportive network. Sharing tales, ideas, and coping methods contributes to a collective strength that eases the journey through perimenopausal transitions.

Adopting a growth mindset during perimenopause is a multifaceted endeavor. Self-acceptance, self-exploration, and dedication to development are essential. A resilient, graceful, and self-empowered person may make it through this transitional period by maintaining a growth mentality, surrounding themselves with good people, and making the most of the chances presented.